STROKE

RECOVER

WORKOUT

A STEP BY STEP GUIDE
On
STROKE RECOVERY WORKOUT

BY
DOCTOR . ANTHONY . WILLIAMS

Table of Contents

INTRODUCTION

UNDERSTANDING STROKE REHABILITATION

Stroke rehabilitation is a critical component of the recovery process for individuals who have experienced a stroke. A stroke, also known as a cerebrovascular accident, occurs when there is a disruption in the blood supply to the brain, resulting in brain cell damage due to lack of oxygen and nutrients. This damage can lead to various physical, cognitive, and emotional impairments, depending on the severity and location of the stroke.

The primary goal of stroke rehabilitation is to help stroke survivors regain as much independence and quality of life as possible. This involves addressing the physical, cognitive, and emotional challenges that may arise following a stroke. Rehabilitation efforts typically begin as soon as the individual's medical condition is stable, often starting in the acute care setting and continuing through various levels of care, including inpatient rehabilitation, outpatient therapy, and home-based programs.

Understanding the principles of stroke rehabilitation is essential for both stroke survivors and their caregivers. Here are some key concepts to consider:

1. **Neuroplasticity**: The brain has the remarkable ability to reorganize and form new neural connections in response to learning, experience, and injury. This concept, known as neuroplasticity, forms the basis of stroke rehabilitation. By engaging in targeted rehabilitation exercises and activities, stroke survivors can promote neuroplasticity and enhance their recovery potential.

2. **Multidisciplinary Approach**: Stroke rehabilitation is often delivered by a multidisciplinary team of healthcare professionals, including physicians, nurses, physical therapists, occupational therapists, speech therapists, and psychologists. Each member of the team plays a unique role in addressing the diverse needs of stroke survivors and maximizing their functional outcomes.

3. **Individualized Care**: Stroke rehabilitation programs should be tailored to meet the specific needs, goals, and abilities of each individual. Factors such as the severity of the stroke, the presence of any comorbidities, and the person's

pre-stroke level of function all influence the rehabilitation process. Personalized treatment plans ensure that interventions are targeted and effective.

4. **Holistic Approach**: Stroke rehabilitation encompasses more than just physical recovery. It also addresses cognitive impairments (such as memory, attention, and executive function deficits) and emotional challenges (such as depression, anxiety, and frustration). A holistic approach to rehabilitation considers the interconnectedness of these domains and promotes overall well-being.

5. **Long-Term Management**: Stroke recovery is often a lifelong journey, and ongoing rehabilitation may be necessary to maintain gains and address new challenges that arise over time. Encouraging continued engagement in rehabilitation activities and promoting a healthy lifestyle can help support long-term recovery and minimize the risk of recurrent strokes.

By understanding the principles and goals of stroke rehabilitation, individuals affected by stroke can actively participate in their recovery journey and work towards optimizing their functional outcomes and quality of life. Effective rehabilitation strategies, combined with support from healthcare professionals and caregivers, play a crucial role in helping stroke survivors rebuild their lives and regain independence.

IMPORTANCE OF EXERCISE IN STROKE RECOVERY

Exercise plays a pivotal role in the rehabilitation process for individuals recovering from a stroke. Stroke, a leading cause of long-term disability worldwide, often results in physical impairments, such as weakness, paralysis, and loss of coordination. Additionally, cognitive and emotional challenges, including memory deficits, depression, and anxiety, can further impact a stroke survivor's ability to function independently.

Incorporating structured exercise programs into stroke rehabilitation offers numerous benefits that can enhance recovery and promote overall well-being. Understanding the importance of exercise in stroke recovery is crucial for both stroke survivors and healthcare professionals alike. Here are several key reasons why exercise is integral to the rehabilitation process:

1. **Physical Rehabilitation**: Stroke survivors often experience impairments in motor function

and mobility due to damage to the brain's motor pathways. Exercise interventions, such as strength training, range of motion exercises, and gait training, help improve muscle strength, flexibility, and coordination. Through targeted exercises, individuals can regain motor control and enhance their ability to perform activities of daily living.

2. **Neuroplasticity and Brain Repair**: Exercise promotes neuroplasticity, the brain's ability to reorganize and form new neural connections in response to learning and experience. Engaging in regular physical activity stimulates the brain's natural repair mechanisms, leading to the formation of new neural pathways that support motor and cognitive recovery. By harnessing the principles of neuroplasticity, exercise can facilitate functional improvements in stroke survivors.

3. **Cardiovascular Health**: Stroke survivors are at an increased risk of cardiovascular complications, including hypertension, high cholesterol, and heart disease. Regular exercise helps improve cardiovascular fitness, lower blood pressure, and reduce the risk of recurrent strokes. Aerobic exercises, such as walking, cycling, and swimming, promote heart health and enhance

overall endurance, contributing to a healthier lifestyle post-stroke.

4. **Functional Independence**: The ability to perform everyday tasks independently is a key indicator of recovery and quality of life for stroke survivors. Exercise programs that focus on activities of daily living (ADLs), such as dressing, grooming, and cooking, help individuals regain functional independence and foster self-confidence. Strengthening exercises targeted at specific functional movements enable stroke survivors to navigate their environment more effectively and participate more fully in social and recreational activities.

5. **Psychological Well-being**: Stroke recovery can be accompanied by emotional challenges, including depression, anxiety, and frustration. Exercise has been shown to have mood-enhancing effects, promoting the release of endorphins and neurotransmitters that improve mood and reduce stress. Participating in regular exercise programs can boost self-esteem, alleviate symptoms of depression, and enhance overall psychological well-being in stroke survivors.

Recognizing the importance of exercise in stroke recovery empowers individuals affected by stroke to actively engage in rehabilitation efforts and maximize their recovery potential. Incorporating exercise into the rehabilitation plan, under the guidance of healthcare professionals, offers a holistic approach to stroke recovery, addressing physical, cognitive, and emotional needs. By prioritizing regular physical activity, stroke survivors can optimize their functional outcomes, improve their quality of life, and embark on a path towards long-term recovery and wellness.

CHAPTER 1

GETTING STARTED

CONSULTATION WITH HEALTHCARE PROVIDER

Before embarking on any exercise program as part of stroke recovery, it is essential for individuals to consult with their healthcare provider. This initial step ensures that the exercise regimen is safe, appropriate, and tailored to the individual's specific needs and abilities. Here's why consultation with a healthcare provider is crucial:

1. **Assessment of Medical History**: Stroke survivors may have pre-existing medical conditions or comorbidities that could impact their ability to engage in certain types of exercise. By consulting with a healthcare provider, individuals can discuss their medical history, including any previous strokes, heart conditions, or other health concerns. This information allows the healthcare provider to make informed recommendations and tailor the exercise program accordingly.

2. **Evaluation of Stroke Severity and Functional Status**: The extent of the stroke and its resulting impairments vary from person to person. Healthcare providers, including physicians, physical therapists, and occupational therapists, can assess the severity of the stroke and evaluate the individual's functional status. This evaluation helps determine the appropriate level of exercise intensity, as well as the types of exercises that are most beneficial for the individual's rehabilitation goals.

3. **Identification of Physical Limitations and Safety Considerations**: Stroke survivors may experience physical limitations, such as muscle weakness, balance deficits, or spasticity, which can impact their ability to engage in certain types of exercise safely. Healthcare providers can identify these limitations and provide guidance on how to adapt exercises to accommodate them. Additionally, they can offer recommendations for assistive devices or modifications to ensure safety during exercise sessions.

4. **Discussion of Goals and Expectations**: Consulting with a healthcare provider allows individuals to discuss their rehabilitation goals and expectations for the exercise program. Whether the

goal is to improve mobility, regain independence in activities of daily living, or enhance overall fitness and well-being, healthcare providers can help set realistic goals and develop a personalized exercise plan to achieve them.

5. **Monitoring Progress and Adjustments**: Regular follow-up appointments with healthcare providers enable ongoing monitoring of progress and adjustments to the exercise program as needed. Healthcare providers can track improvements in physical function, address any challenges or concerns that arise during the rehabilitation process, and make modifications to the exercise regimen to optimize outcomes.

6. **Integration with Comprehensive Rehabilitation Plan**: Exercise is just one component of stroke rehabilitation, which may also include other interventions such as physical therapy, occupational therapy, speech therapy, and medication management. Consulting with a healthcare provider ensures that the exercise program is integrated seamlessly with the overall rehabilitation plan, maximizing the effectiveness of treatment and promoting holistic recovery.

In summary, consultation with a healthcare provider is a critical first step in getting started with exercise as part of stroke recovery. By working closely with healthcare professionals, individuals can receive personalized guidance, support, and supervision throughout the rehabilitation process, ultimately leading to improved functional outcomes and enhanced quality of life.

ASSESSING PHYSICAL ABILITIES AND LIMITATIONS
Before initiating an exercise program for stroke recovery, it is essential to assess the individual's physical abilities and limitations. This assessment provides valuable information that guides the development of a safe and effective exercise regimen tailored to the individual's specific needs. Here's how to assess physical abilities and limitations:

1. **Range of Motion (ROM) Assessment**: Begin by evaluating the individual's range of motion in various joints, including the shoulders, elbows, wrists, hips, knees, and ankles. Determine if there are any restrictions or limitations in movement due to muscle weakness, spasticity, or contractures resulting from the stroke. Assessing ROM helps

identify areas that may require targeted stretching exercises to improve flexibility and mobility.

2. **Strength Assessment**: Assess muscle strength in both the affected and unaffected limbs using standardized strength testing protocols. This evaluation helps identify weakness and asymmetries, which are common after a stroke. Pay particular attention to muscle groups involved in functional tasks such as standing, walking, reaching, and gripping. Strength assessments can guide the selection of appropriate strengthening exercises to address muscle imbalances and improve overall functional capacity.

3. **Balance and Coordination Assessment**: Evaluate the individual's balance and coordination abilities to identify deficits that may impact mobility and stability. Use standardized balance tests, such as the Berg Balance Scale or Timed Up and Go test, to assess static and dynamic balance. Observe the individual's ability to maintain postural stability, shift weight, and perform coordinated movements. Balance and coordination assessments inform the development of exercises aimed at improving balance control and reducing the risk of falls.

4. **Functional Mobility Assessment**: Assess the individual's ability to perform activities of daily living (ADLs) independently, such as dressing, grooming, toileting, and transferring in and out of bed or chairs. Observe how the individual moves and interacts with their environment to identify specific challenges or limitations. Functional mobility assessments provide insight into the individual's level of independence and help prioritize rehabilitation goals related to functional tasks.

5. **Cardiovascular Fitness Assessment**: Evaluate cardiovascular fitness and endurance using standardized tests, such as the six-minute walk test or the graded exercise test. Assess the individual's ability to sustain aerobic activity and monitor heart rate response to exercise. Cardiovascular fitness assessments help gauge the individual's tolerance for physical activity and guide the prescription of appropriate aerobic exercises to improve cardiovascular health and stamina.

6. **Assistive Device Assessment**: Determine if the individual requires assistive devices or adaptive equipment to facilitate mobility and participation in exercise activities. Assess the use of mobility aids such as canes, walkers, wheelchairs, or orthotic

devices and ensure proper fit and function. Assistive device assessments help optimize safety and mobility during exercise sessions and promote independence in daily life.

By thoroughly assessing the individual's physical abilities and limitations, healthcare professionals can develop a personalized exercise program that addresses specific rehabilitation goals and promotes functional recovery following a stroke. Regular reassessment of physical function allows for adjustments to the exercise regimen as the individual progresses through the rehabilitation process, ultimately optimizing outcomes and enhancing quality of life.

SETTING REALISTIC GOALS
Setting realistic goals is a crucial step in initiating an exercise program for stroke recovery. Realistic goals provide a clear direction for rehabilitation efforts, motivate individuals to stay committed to their exercise regimen, and serve as benchmarks for tracking progress over time. Here are some key considerations for setting realistic goals:

1. **Understand the Individual's Needs and Abilities**: Begin by gaining a thorough understanding of the individual's unique needs,

abilities, and limitations. Consider factors such as the severity of the stroke, the extent of physical impairments, cognitive function, and pre-stroke level of activity. Tailor goals to align with the individual's current abilities while challenging them to make meaningful improvements.

2. **Identify Specific Areas for Improvement**: Collaborate with the individual and their healthcare team to identify specific areas for improvement based on the results of physical assessments and functional evaluations. Focus on addressing deficits in strength, range of motion, balance, coordination, mobility, and cardiovascular fitness. Setting specific, measurable goals ensures clarity and accountability throughout the rehabilitation process.

3. **Establish Short-Term and Long-Term Goals**: Break down larger rehabilitation objectives into smaller, achievable milestones to facilitate progress and maintain motivation. Set short-term goals that can be accomplished within a few weeks or months, as well as long-term goals that represent the desired outcome of the rehabilitation program. Short-term goals provide immediate feedback and reinforcement, while long-term goals provide a sense of purpose and direction.

4. **Use the SMART Goal Framework**: Apply the SMART criteria—Specific, Measurable, Achievable, Relevant, and Time-bound—to ensure that goals are well-defined and attainable. For example, instead of setting a vague goal like "improve walking ability," a SMART goal might be "increase walking distance from 50 meters to 100 meters within three months." SMART goals provide clarity and focus, guiding individuals toward success.

5. **Consider Personal Preferences and Motivations**: Take into account the individual's interests, preferences, and motivations when setting goals to enhance engagement and adherence to the exercise program. Incorporate activities that the individual enjoys or finds meaningful, whether it's walking in nature, participating in group exercise classes, or pursuing hobbies that promote physical activity. Aligning goals with personal interests increases intrinsic motivation and fosters a sense of ownership over the rehabilitation process.

6. **Monitor Progress and Adjust Goals as Needed**: Continuously monitor progress towards achieving goals and adjust them as necessary based on the individual's evolving needs and capabilities. Celebrate achievements and milestones along the

way to maintain motivation and reinforce positive behavior. Be flexible in modifying goals to accommodate setbacks or changes in circumstances, while remaining focused on the ultimate objective of maximizing functional independence and quality of life.

By setting realistic goals that are tailored to the individual's needs, abilities, and preferences, healthcare professionals can empower stroke survivors to actively participate in their rehabilitation journey and work towards meaningful outcomes. Clear, achievable goals provide a roadmap for success, guiding individuals through the stages of recovery and ultimately leading to improved physical function, confidence, and overall well-being.

CHAPTER 2

WARM-UP EXERCISES

RANGE OF MOTION EXERCISES
Range of motion (ROM) exercises are an essential component of any warm-up routine, especially for individuals recovering from a stroke. These exercises help improve flexibility, increase joint mobility, and reduce the risk of injury during subsequent physical activity. Range of motion exercises target specific muscle groups and joints, promoting circulation and preparing the body for more strenuous exercise. Here are some effective range of motion exercises for stroke recovery warm-up routines:

1. **Neck Rotations**:
   - Sit or stand comfortably with the spine tall and shoulders relaxed.
   - Slowly turn the head to one side, bringing the chin towards the shoulder.
   - Hold the stretch for 10-15 seconds, feeling a gentle stretch along the side of the neck.
   - Return to the starting position and repeat on the opposite side.

- Perform 5-10 repetitions on each side, gradually increasing the range of motion as tolerated.

2. **Shoulder Circles**:
   - Begin with the arms at the sides and the elbows slightly bent.
   - Slowly rotate the shoulders in a circular motion, bringing the shoulders forward, up towards the ears, back, and down.
   - Perform 5-10 circles in a forward direction, then reverse the motion and perform 5-10 circles in a backward direction.
   - Focus on maintaining smooth, controlled movements and gradually increase the size of the circles as flexibility improves.

3. **Arm Swings**:
   - Stand with feet shoulder-width apart and arms relaxed at the sides.
   - Swing both arms forward and upward, reaching towards the ceiling.
   - Continue the motion, swinging the arms back and down behind the body.
   - Repeat for 10-15 repetitions, allowing the arms to swing freely and gradually increasing the range of motion with each swing.

4. **Wrist Flexion and Extension**:
   - Extend one arm in front of the body with the palm facing down.
   - Use the opposite hand to gently press down on the fingers, stretching the wrist and forearm.
   - Hold the stretch for 10-15 seconds, then release and repeat on the other side.
   - Next, extend the arm with the palm facing up and gently press down on the back of the hand, stretching the wrist in the opposite direction.
   - Hold for 10-15 seconds and repeat on the other side.
   - Perform 5-10 repetitions of each stretch to improve wrist flexibility and range of motion.

5. **Ankle Circles**:
   - Sit or lie down comfortably with one leg extended.
   - Rotate the ankle in a circular motion, moving the foot clockwise and then counterclockwise.
   - Perform 10-15 circles in each direction, focusing on moving through the full range of motion.
   - Switch to the other leg and repeat the exercise to loosen up the ankles and improve mobility.

6. **Knee Extensions**:
   - Sit on a chair with feet flat on the floor.

- Straighten one leg out in front of you, keeping the foot flexed.
- Hold the position for a few seconds, feeling a stretch in the back of the thigh.
- Return the foot to the starting position and repeat on the other side.
- Perform 5-10 repetitions on each leg to improve knee flexibility and range of motion.

Performing a range of motion exercises as part of a warm-up routine helps prepare the body for more strenuous activity while promoting flexibility and joint mobility. It's essential to perform these exercises gently and gradually increase the range of motion over time to avoid overstretching or causing discomfort. Incorporating a range of motion exercises into a regular warm-up routine can contribute to improved physical function and overall well-being during stroke recovery.

GENTLE STRETCHING ROUTINE
A gentle stretching routine is an integral part of any warm-up regimen, particularly for individuals recovering from a stroke. Stretching helps improve flexibility, reduce muscle tension, and enhance joint mobility, preparing the body for subsequent physical activity. Incorporating gentle stretching exercises into a warm-up routine can help increase

circulation, loosen tight muscles, and promote relaxation. Here are some effective gentle stretching exercises for stroke recovery warm-ups:

1. **Neck Stretch**:
   - Sit or stand tall with the shoulders relaxed.
   - Gently tilt the head to one side, bringing the ear towards the shoulder.
   - Hold the stretch for 15-30 seconds, feeling a gentle stretch along the side of the neck.
   - Return to the starting position and repeat on the opposite side.
   - Perform 2-3 repetitions on each side, focusing on maintaining smooth, controlled movements.

2. **Shoulder Stretch**:
   - Stand or sit comfortably with the spine tall and shoulders relaxed.
   - Reach one arm across the chest, using the opposite hand to gently press the arm towards the body.
   - Hold the stretch for 15-30 seconds, feeling a gentle stretch in the shoulder and upper back.
   - Release the stretch and repeat on the other side.
   - Perform 2-3 repetitions on each side, gradually increasing the stretch as tolerated.

3. **Chest Opener Stretch**:
   - Stand with feet hip-width apart and arms relaxed at the sides.
   - Interlace the fingers behind the back, straightening the arms and gently lifting the chest.
   - Hold the stretch for 15-30 seconds, feeling a gentle opening in the chest and shoulders.
   - Release the stretch and repeat as desired, focusing on maintaining relaxed breathing throughout.

4. **Hamstring Stretch**:
   - Sit on the floor with one leg extended and the other leg bent.
   - Gently lean forward from the hips, reaching towards the extended leg.
   - Hold the stretch for 15-30 seconds, feeling a gentle stretch in the back of the thigh.
   - Repeat on the other side, alternating between legs for 2-3 repetitions on each side.

5. **Quadriceps Stretch**:
   - Stand tall with feet hip-width apart and hold onto a stable surface for balance if needed.
   - Bend one knee and bring the heel towards the buttocks, grasping the ankle or foot with the hand.
   - Gently pull the heel towards the buttocks, feeling a stretch in the front of the thigh.

- Hold the stretch for 15-30 seconds, then release and repeat on the other side.
   - Perform 2-3 repetitions on each leg, focusing on maintaining proper alignment and avoiding excessive strain.

6. **Calf Stretch**:
   - Stand facing a wall with one foot forward and the other foot back.
   - Lean forward, placing both hands on the wall for support, and bend the front knee.
   - Keep the back leg straight and press the heel into the floor, feeling a stretch in the calf muscle.
   - Hold the stretch for 15-30 seconds, then switch legs and repeat on the other side.
   - Perform 2-3 repetitions on each leg, gradually increasing the intensity of the stretch as tolerated.

Performing a gentle stretching routine as part of a warm-up helps prepare the muscles and joints for physical activity while promoting relaxation and reducing the risk of injury. It's essential to stretch gently and avoid bouncing or jerking movements, especially for individuals recovering from a stroke. Incorporating these stretching exercises into a regular warm-up routine can contribute to improved flexibility, mobility, and overall well-being during stroke recovery.

BREATHING EXERCISES

Breathing exercises are an integral part of any warm-up routine, particularly for individuals undergoing stroke recovery. These exercises help enhance lung function, increase oxygen flow to the muscles, and promote relaxation, which can be beneficial before engaging in more strenuous physical activity. Breathing exercises also provide an opportunity to focus on mindfulness and centering the mind-body connection. Here are some gentle breathing exercises suitable for warm-up routines:

1. **Diaphragmatic Breathing**:
   - Sit or lie down comfortably with your spine tall and shoulders relaxed.
   - Place one hand on your abdomen and the other hand on your chest.
   - Inhale deeply through your nose, allowing your abdomen to expand as you fill your lungs with air.
   - Exhale slowly through your mouth, drawing your navel towards your spine and feeling your abdomen deflate.
   - Focus on breathing deeply into your diaphragm, rather than shallow chest breathing.
   - Repeat for several breaths, gradually increasing the length of each inhale and exhale.

2. **Pursed Lip Breathing**:
   - Sit comfortably with your spine tall and shoulders relaxed.
   - Inhale slowly and deeply through your nose for a count of two.
   - Pucker your lips as if you're going to blow out a candle.
   - Exhale slowly and gently through pursed lips for a count of four, allowing the breath to escape slowly.
   - Focus on making the exhale twice as long as the inhale, promoting relaxation and stress reduction.
   - Repeat for several breaths, maintaining a smooth and steady rhythm.

3. **Alternate Nostril Breathing**:
   - Sit comfortably with your spine tall and shoulders relaxed.
   - Use your right thumb to close your right nostril and inhale deeply through your left nostril.
   - Close your left nostril with your right ring finger and exhale slowly through your right nostril.
   - Inhale deeply through your right nostril, then close it with your right thumb and exhale through your left nostril.
   - Continue alternating nostrils for several breaths, focusing on the sensation of air moving in and out of each nostril.

- This technique promotes balance and relaxation
in the body and mind.

4. **Box Breathing**:
   - Sit or lie down comfortably with your spine tall
and shoulders relaxed.
   - Inhale deeply through your nose for a count of
four, feeling your abdomen rise.
   - Hold your breath for a count of four,
maintaining a steady pause without straining.
   - Exhale slowly through your mouth for a count of
four, allowing your abdomen to fall.
   - Hold your breath out for a count of four before
inhaling again to complete the cycle.
   - Repeat for several rounds, focusing on
maintaining a smooth and steady rhythm.

5. **Mindful Breathing**:
   - Sit or lie down comfortably with your spine tall
and shoulders relaxed.
   - Close your eyes and bring your awareness to
your breath, noticing the sensation of air flowing in
and out of your body.
   - Take slow, deep breaths, allowing each inhale to
fill your lungs completely and each exhale to release
tension and stress.

- With each breath, imagine sending oxygen and relaxation to any areas of tension or discomfort in your body.
- Focus on the present moment, letting go of any distractions or worries, and simply being with your breath.
- Continue for several minutes, allowing yourself to feel calm, centered, and grounded.

Incorporating breathing exercises into a warm-up routine before engaging in physical activity can help prepare the body and mind, promote relaxation, and enhance overall well-being during stroke recovery. These gentle exercises can be performed anywhere, anytime, making them a convenient and effective addition to daily self-care practices.

CHAPTER 3

STRENGTH BUILDING EXERCISES

UPPER BODY STRENGTHENING EXERCISES

Upper body strengthening exercises are vital for improving arm function, shoulder stability, and overall upper body strength in individuals undergoing stroke recovery. These exercises target the muscles of the arms, shoulders, chest, and upper back, helping to regain functional abilities such as reaching, lifting, and carrying objects. Here are some effective upper body strengthening exercises suitable for stroke recovery:

1. **Assisted Shoulder Flexion**:
   - Sit or stand with good posture, holding a resistance band or towel in both hands.
   - Begin with the arms by the sides, palms facing inward.
   - Slowly raise both arms overhead, keeping them straight and in line with the shoulders.
   - Lower the arms back down to the starting position with control.

- Repeat for 10-15 repetitions, gradually
increasing resistance as strength improves.

2. **Seated Rows**:
  - Sit on a chair or bench with a resistance band
anchored in front of you at chest height.
  - Grasp the ends of the band with both hands,
palms facing inward.
  - Keeping the elbows close to the body, pull the
band towards your chest, squeezing the shoulder
blades together.
  - Slowly return to the starting position,
maintaining tension in the band.
  - Perform 10-15 repetitions, focusing on engaging
the muscles of the upper back.

3. **Bicep Curls**:
  - Sit or stand with good posture, holding a
dumbbell or resistance band in each hand, palms
facing forward.
  - Keep the elbows close to the body and slowly
curl the weights towards the shoulders, contracting
the biceps.
  - Pause briefly at the top of the movement, then
lower the weights back down with control.
  - Perform 10-15 repetitions, gradually increasing
the weight or resistance as strength improves.

4. **Tricep Extensions**:
   - Sit or stand with good posture, holding a dumbbell or resistance band in one hand, arm raised overhead.
   - Bend the elbow, lowering the weight behind the head until the forearm is parallel to the floor.
   - Extend the elbow, straightening the arm and lifting the weight back up towards the ceiling.
   - Perform 10-15 repetitions on each arm, focusing on keeping the upper arm stable and engaging the triceps.

5. **Wall Push-Ups**:
   - Stand facing a wall with arms extended, hands flat against the wall at shoulder height and slightly wider than shoulder-width apart.
   - Keeping the body in a straight line from head to heels, bend the elbows and lower the chest towards the wall.
   - Push through the palms to straighten the arms and return to the starting position.
   - Perform 10-15 repetitions, focusing on maintaining proper alignment and engaging the chest and arm muscles.

6. **Shoulder External Rotation**:
   - Sit or stand with good posture, holding a resistance band in front of you at waist height.
   - Grasp one end of the band with the hand of the affected side, keeping the elbow bent to 90 degrees and the forearm parallel to the floor.
   - Rotate the forearm outward, away from the body, against the resistance of the band.
   - Slowly return to the starting position with control.
   - Perform 10-15 repetitions on each side, focusing on strengthening the muscles involved in shoulder external rotation.

It's essential to start with light resistance and gradually increase the intensity as strength improves. Perform these exercises 2-3 times per week, aiming for 1-3 sets of 10-15 repetitions for each exercise. Consistency and proper form are key to maximizing the benefits of upper body strengthening exercises during stroke recovery.

LOWER BODY STRENGTHENING EXERCISES

Lower body strengthening exercises are essential for improving mobility, stability, and overall lower body strength in individuals undergoing stroke recovery. These exercises target the muscles of the legs, hips, and core, helping to enhance balance, walking ability, and independence in daily activities. Here are some effective lower body strengthening exercises suitable for stroke recovery:

1. **Chair Squats**:
   - Begin by sitting in a sturdy chair with feet hip-width apart and arms crossed over the chest.
   - Engage the core muscles and slowly stand up, pushing through the heels and keeping the back straight.
   - Lower back down to the seated position with control, aiming to tap the buttocks lightly on the chair.
   - Perform 10-15 repetitions, gradually increasing the depth of the squat as strength improves.

2. **Leg Raises**:
   - Lie on your back with legs extended and arms by your sides.
   - Lift one leg off the floor, keeping it straight and engaging the muscles of the thigh and hip.
   - Hold for a few seconds, then lower the leg back down with control.
   - Repeat on the other side, alternating legs for 10-15 repetitions on each side.

3. **Standing Calf Raises**:
   - Stand upright with feet hip-width apart and hands resting on a stable surface for support, such as a wall or countertop.
   - Rise up onto the balls of the feet, lifting the heels as high as possible.
   - Hold for a few seconds at the top, then lower the heels back down to the ground.
   - Perform 10-15 repetitions, focusing on engaging the calf muscles and maintaining balance.

4. **Step-Ups**:
   - Stand in front of a step or sturdy platform with feet hip-width apart.
   - Step one foot onto the platform, pressing through the heel to lift the body up.
   - Bring the opposite foot up to meet the first foot on the platform.
   - Step back down with the same foot, followed by the other foot.
   - Repeat, alternating legs for 10-15 repetitions on each side, gradually increasing the height of the step as strength improves.

5. **Seated Leg Press**:
   - Sit in a chair with feet flat on the floor and knees bent at a 90-degree angle.

- Place a resistance band around the balls of the feet, holding the ends of the band in each hand.
- Push the feet forward, extending the legs and straightening the knees against the resistance of the band.
- Slowly return to the starting position with control.
- Perform 10-15 repetitions, focusing on engaging the muscles of the thighs and hips.

6. **Hip Abduction/Adduction**:
- Sit in a chair with feet flat on the floor and knees bent.
- Place a small ball or rolled-up towel between the knees.
- Squeeze the knees together, engaging the inner thigh muscles.
- Hold for a few seconds, then release and repeat for 10-15 repetitions.
- Next, sit with legs extended and feet slightly apart.
- Place a resistance band around both ankles and gently push the legs outward against the resistance of the band.
- Hold for a few seconds, then release and repeat for 10-15 repetitions, focusing on engaging the muscles of the outer thighs and hips.

It's essential to start with light resistance and gradually increase the intensity as strength improves. Perform these exercises 2-3 times per week, aiming for 1-3 sets of 10-15 repetitions for each exercise. Consistency and proper form are key to maximizing the benefits of lower body strengthening exercises during stroke recovery.

CORE STRENGTHENING EXERCISES
Core strengthening exercises are fundamental for individuals undergoing stroke recovery as they help improve stability, balance, and posture. A strong core also supports everyday movements and reduces the risk of falls. Here are some effective core strengthening exercises suitable for stroke recovery:

1. **Seated Marching**:
   - Sit upright in a chair with feet flat on the floor.
   - Lift one foot off the floor, bringing the knee towards the chest.
   - Lower the foot back down and repeat with the opposite leg.
   - Continue alternating legs in a marching motion for 10-15 repetitions on each side, engaging the core to maintain balance and stability.

2. **Seated Twists**:
   - Sit upright in a chair with feet flat on the floor and hands clasped together in front of the chest.
   - Rotate the torso to one side, twisting from the waist while keeping the hips and legs stable.
   - Return to the center and twist to the other side, alternating sides for 10-15 repetitions.
   - Focus on engaging the oblique muscles along the sides of the torso and maintaining good posture throughout the movement.

3. **Bridge**:
   - Lie on your back with knees bent and feet flat on the floor, hip-width apart.
   - Engage the core and glutes, then lift the hips off the floor until the body forms a straight line from shoulders to knees.
   - Hold the bridge position for a few seconds, then lower the hips back down with control.
   - Repeat for 10-15 repetitions, focusing on maintaining stability and avoiding arching the lower back.

4. **Plank**:
   - Start in a kneeling position on the floor with hands shoulder-width apart.

- Extend the legs behind you, coming into a plank
position with the body forming a straight line from
head to heels.
   - Engage the core muscles and hold the plank
position for 10-30 seconds, depending on your level
of strength and stability.
   - Focus on keeping the hips level and avoiding
sagging or lifting the hips too high.

5. **Dead Bug**:
   - Lie on your back with knees bent and arms
extended towards the ceiling.
   - Engage the core muscles and slowly lower one
arm and the opposite leg towards the floor,
maintaining contact with the ground.
   - Return to the starting position and repeat on the
opposite side.
   - Continue alternating sides for 10-15 repetitions,
focusing on maintaining stability and control.

6. **Side Plank**:
   - Lie on your side with legs extended and feet
stacked on top of each other.
   - Prop yourself up on your forearm, elbow directly
beneath the shoulder, and lift your hips off the
floor, creating a straight line from head to heels.

- Engage the core muscles and hold the side plank position for 10-30 seconds, then switch sides and repeat.
- Focus on keeping the body in a straight line and avoiding sagging or sinking into the shoulder.

Perform these core strengthening exercises 2-3 times per week, aiming for 1-3 sets of 10-15 repetitions for each exercise. Start with modifications or assistance as needed and gradually progress to more challenging variations as strength improves. Consistency and proper form are essential for maximizing the benefits of core strengthening during stroke recovery.

CHAPTER 4

BALANCE AND COORDINATION EXERCISES

STATIC BALANCE EXERCISES
Static balance exercises are essential for improving stability and reducing the risk of falls in individuals undergoing stroke recovery. These exercises focus on maintaining equilibrium while standing still, helping to strengthen the muscles involved in balance and improving proprioception. Here are some effective static balance exercises suitable for stroke recovery:

1. **Tandem Stance**:
   - Stand with one foot directly in front of the other, heel to toe, maintaining a narrow base of support.
   - Keep the arms by your sides or place hands on hips for stability.
   - Focus on maintaining your balance and holding the position for 10-30 seconds.
   - Switch feet and repeat the exercise, aiming to improve balance on both sides.

2. **Single-Leg Stance**:
   - Stand on one leg with the knee slightly bent and the opposite foot lifted off the floor.
   - Keep the standing leg straight but not locked, and engage the core muscles for stability.
   - Hold the position for 10-30 seconds, maintaining balance and control.
   - Switch legs and repeat the exercise, aiming to improve balance on both sides.

3. **Weight Shifts**:
   - Stand with feet hip-width apart and arms relaxed at your sides.
   - Slowly shift your weight onto one leg while lifting the opposite foot off the floor slightly.
   - Hold the position for a few seconds, then return to the starting position.
   - Repeat the weight shift to the opposite side, focusing on maintaining balance and control.
   - Perform 10-15 repetitions on each side, gradually increasing the range of motion as balance improves.

4. **Clock Reach**:
   - Imagine yourself standing in the center of a clock face, with 12 o'clock directly in front of you and 6 o'clock behind you.

- Lift one foot off the floor and reach forward with the opposite hand to touch the imaginary numbers on the clock face.
- Return to the starting position and repeat the reach in different directions, including forward, to the sides, and diagonally.
- Focus on maintaining balance and control throughout the movement, engaging the core muscles to stabilize the body.
- Perform 5-10 hits on each side, gradually increasing the challenge by reaching further or holding the position for longer.

5. **Stork Stand**:
- Stand on one leg with the knee slightly bent and the opposite foot lifted off the floor.
- Extend the arms out to the sides for balance, or place hands on hips if preferred.
- Hold the position for 10-30 seconds, maintaining balance and stability.
- Switch legs and repeat the exercise, aiming to improve balance on both sides.

6. **Eyes Closed Balance**:
- Stand with feet hip-width apart and arms relaxed at your sides.

- Close your eyes and focus on maintaining your balance without visual input.
   - Hold the position for 10-30 seconds, relying on proprioception and kinesthetic awareness to stay upright.
   - Open your eyes and return to the starting position, repeating the exercise as desired to challenge balance further.

Perform these static balance exercises 2-3 times per week, aiming for 1-3 sets of 10-30 seconds for each exercise. Start with assistance or support as needed and gradually progress to more challenging variations as balance improves. Consistency and proper technique are key to maximizing the benefits of static balance exercises during stroke recovery.

DYNAMIC BALANCE EXERCISES

Dynamic balance exercises are crucial for improving stability and coordination in individuals undergoing stroke recovery. These exercises involve movement while maintaining equilibrium, helping to strengthen muscles, enhance proprioception, and reduce the risk of falls. Here are some effective dynamic balance exercises suitable for stroke recovery:

1. **Leg Swings**:
   - Stand near a sturdy support, such as a wall or chair, for balance if needed.
   - Swing one leg forward and backward in a controlled motion, keeping the torso upright and maintaining balance on the supporting leg.
   - Perform 10-15 swings on each leg, gradually increasing the range of motion as balance improves.
   - Repeat the exercise with side-to-side leg swings, swinging the leg out to the side and back towards the midline.

2. **Heel-to-Toe Walk**:
   - Begin by standing with the heel of one foot touching the toes of the other foot, creating a straight line.
   - Take small steps forward, placing the heel of one foot directly in front of the toes of the opposite foot with each step.
   - Focus on maintaining balance and coordination while walking in a straight line.
   - Continue for 10-20 steps, then turn around and walk back in the opposite direction.
   - Gradually increase the distance walked as balance and confidence improve.

3. **Step-Ups with Knee Lift**:
   - Stand in front of a step or platform with feet hip-width apart.

- Step up onto the platform with one foot,
bringing the opposite knee up towards the chest.
- Balance on the stepping foot for a moment, then
step back down with control.
- Repeat the exercise on the same side for 10-15
repetitions, then switch legs and repeat on the other
side.
- Focus on maintaining stability and control
throughout the movement, engaging the core
muscles for balance.

4. **Crossover Steps**:
- Stand with feet hip-width apart and arms
relaxed at your sides.
- Take a diagonal step forward and across the
body with one foot, crossing over the midline.
- Follow with the opposite foot, stepping behind
and to the side of the lead foot.
- Continue alternating crossover steps, moving
forward or backward as space allows.
- Focus on maintaining balance and coordination
while crossing the midline with each step.

5. **Lateral Side Steps**:
- Stand with feet together and knees slightly bent,
holding onto a stable support if needed for balance.

- Take a step to the side with one foot, keeping the knees bent and the torso upright.
   - Follow with the opposite foot, bringing the feet back together.
   - Continue side-stepping in one direction for 10-15 steps, then switch directions and repeat.
   - Focus on maintaining balance and control while moving laterally.

6. **Balance Board Exercises**:
   - Stand on a balance board or wobble board with feet hip-width apart, holding onto a support if needed for stability.
   - Engage the core muscles and shift your weight to maintain balance on the board.
   - Experiment with different movements, such as rocking side to side, front to back, or in circles.
   - Gradually increase the challenge by closing your eyes or performing exercises with one leg lifted.

Perform these dynamic balance exercises 2-3 times per week, aiming for 1-3 sets of 10-15 repetitions for each exercise. Start with assistance or support as needed and gradually progress to more challenging variations as balance and coordination improve. Consistency and proper technique are essential for maximizing the benefits of dynamic balance exercises during stroke recovery.

COORDINATION DRILLS

Coordination drills are valuable for enhancing motor skills, agility, and proprioception in individuals undergoing stroke recovery. These exercises focus on improving the ability to perform coordinated movements and maintain balance while engaging in various activities. Here are some effective coordination drills suitable for stroke recovery:

1. **Crossover Marching**:
   - Stand with feet hip-width apart and arms relaxed at your sides.
   - Lift one knee towards the opposite elbow, crossing the midline of the body.
   - Return the foot to the ground and repeat with the opposite knee and elbow.
   - Continue alternating crossover marches, focusing on coordinating movement between the upper and lower body.

2. **Figure 8 Drill**:
   - Set up two cones or markers several feet apart on the floor.
   - Stand behind one cone and begin moving in a figure-eight pattern around both cones.
   - Step over and around each cone, maintaining a steady pace and fluid movement.

- Focus on coordinating footwork and shifting weight smoothly between turns.

3. **Box Drill**:
  - Create a square outline on the floor with tape or markers, approximately 2-3 feet wide.
  - Stand at one corner of the square and move in a clockwise direction, stepping into each corner of the box.
  - Step forward, sideways, backward, and sideways again, completing one lap around the box.
  - Repeat the drill in a counterclockwise direction, focusing on maintaining balance and control while changing direction.

4. **Agility Ladder Drills**:
  - Lay an agility ladder flat on the floor or create a makeshift ladder with tape or chalk.
  - Perform a variety of agility ladder drills, such as high knees, lateral shuffles, and grapevine steps.
  - Focus on stepping quickly and accurately through the ladder rungs, coordinating footwork and maintaining balance.

5. **Ball Toss and Catch**:
   - Stand facing a partner or a wall with a small ball in hand.
   - Toss the ball back and forth between hands, varying the height and trajectory of the throw.
   - Challenge coordination by tossing the ball with one hand while simultaneously catching with the other hand.
   - Focus on tracking the ball with your eyes, coordinating hand movements, and maintaining balance while catching and throwing.

6. **Mirror Drill**:
   - Stand facing a partner with enough space between you to move freely.
   - Take turns mirroring each other's movements, such as stepping forward, sideways, or rotating.
   - The leader performs a sequence of movements while the follower attempts to replicate the actions as closely as possible.
   - Focus on coordinating movements and maintaining balance while matching your partner's actions.

Perform these coordination drills 2-3 times per week, aiming for 1-3 sets of 10-15 repetitions for each exercise. Start with slow, controlled movements and gradually increase speed and complexity as coordination improves. Consistency and practice are key to maximizing the benefits of coordination drills during stroke recovery.

CHAPTER 5

CARDIOVASCULAR CONDITIONING

LOW-IMPACT AEROBIC EXERCISES
Low-impact aerobic exercises are essential for improving cardiovascular health, endurance, and overall fitness in individuals undergoing stroke recovery. These exercises provide a cardiovascular workout without placing excessive stress on the joints, making them suitable for individuals with mobility challenges or joint pain. Low-impact aerobic exercises help increase heart rate, improve circulation, and boost energy levels while minimizing the risk of injury. Here are some effective low-impact aerobic exercises suitable for stroke recovery:

1. **Walking**:
   - Walking is a simple yet effective low-impact aerobic exercise that can be tailored to individual fitness levels.
   - Start with short walks at a comfortable pace, gradually increasing duration and intensity as tolerated.

- Use a treadmill with handrails for added stability or walk outdoors in a safe, flat environment such as a park or walking path.

2. **Cycling**:
   - Stationary cycling or using a recumbent bike is an excellent low-impact aerobic exercise option for stroke recovery.
   - Adjust the resistance and speed to match individual fitness levels and gradually increase intensity over time.
   - Cycling strengthens the lower body muscles, improves cardiovascular fitness, and enhances range of motion in the hips and knees.

3. **Elliptical Trainer**:
   - The elliptical trainer provides a low-impact, full-body workout that engages both the upper and lower body muscles.
   - Adjust the resistance and incline settings to customize the intensity of the workout.
   - Focus on maintaining proper posture and using smooth, controlled movements to minimize strain on the joints.

4. **Water Aerobics**:
   - Water aerobics is an excellent low-impact exercise option that provides resistance while minimizing stress on the joints.
   - Perform a variety of movements, such as walking, jogging, kicking, and arm exercises, in chest-deep water.
   - Water buoyancy supports the body, making it easier to move and reducing the risk of injury.

5. **Rowing Machine**:
   - The rowing machine provides a low-impact, full-body cardiovascular workout that strengthens the arms, legs, and core muscles.
   - Focus on maintaining proper form and using smooth, controlled strokes to avoid strain on the back or shoulders.
   - Adjust the resistance and speed settings to match individual fitness levels and gradually increase intensity over time.

6. **Dancing**:
   - Dancing is a fun and enjoyable low-impact aerobic exercise that can be adapted to suit various fitness levels and preferences.
   - Choose dance styles such as ballroom, salsa, or Zumba, which incorporate rhythmic movements

and music to elevate heart rate and improve cardiovascular fitness.

- Follow along with instructional dance videos or join a dance class tailored to individuals with mobility challenges or disabilities.

Perform low-impact aerobic exercises for at least 20-30 minutes, 3-5 days per week, to reap the cardiovascular benefits. Start with shorter durations and gradually increase duration and intensity as fitness improves. Always consult with a healthcare professional before starting a new exercise program, especially if you have underlying health conditions or concerns. Consistency and gradual progression are key to maximizing the cardiovascular benefits of low-impact aerobic exercises during stroke recovery.

AQUATIC THERAPY

Aquatic therapy, also known as water therapy or hydrotherapy, is a highly beneficial form of cardiovascular conditioning for individuals undergoing stroke recovery. Utilizing the buoyancy and resistance of water, aquatic therapy provides a safe and supportive environment for cardiovascular exercise while minimizing stress on the joints and muscles. Here's why aquatic therapy is effective and how it can be incorporated into a stroke recovery regimen:

Benefits of Aquatic Therapy:

1. **Low-Impact Exercise:** Water provides buoyancy, which reduces the impact on joints and allows for gentle movement, making aquatic therapy suitable for individuals with mobility challenges or joint pain.

2. **Muscle Strengthening:** Water resistance provides natural resistance against movement, helping to strengthen muscles throughout the body, including the arms, legs, and core.

3. **Improved Range of Motion:** The buoyancy of water supports the body and reduces the effects of gravity, allowing for increased range of motion in joints and muscles, which is especially beneficial for individuals with spasticity or stiffness after a stroke.

4. **Enhanced Circulation:** The hydrostatic pressure of water helps improve circulation, reducing swelling and promoting healing in injured tissues.

5. **Balance and Coordination:** Aquatic therapy challenges balance and coordination as individuals navigate through the water, helping to improve proprioception and stability.

6. **Cardiovascular Fitness:** Engaging in aerobic activities in the water, such as walking or swimming, increases heart rate and improves cardiovascular endurance without placing undue stress on the cardiovascular system.

Incorporating Aquatic Therapy into Stroke Recovery:

1. **Consultation with Healthcare Provider:** Before starting aquatic therapy, it's essential to consult with a healthcare provider or physical therapist to ensure it's safe and appropriate for your individual condition and needs.

2. **Professional Supervision:** Work with a qualified aquatic therapist or physical therapist who has experience working with individuals recovering from stroke. They can create a customized aquatic therapy program tailored to your specific goals and abilities.

3. **Warm-Up Exercises:** Begin each aquatic therapy session with gentle warm-up exercises to prepare the body for activity and reduce the risk of injury. This may include walking or jogging in place, arm circles, and gentle stretching.

4. **Aerobic Activities:** Incorporate aerobic activities into your aquatic therapy routine to improve cardiovascular fitness. This may include walking or jogging in the water, swimming laps, or using water resistance equipment such as aquatic dumbbells.

5. **Strength Training:** Use the resistance of water to perform strength training exercises targeting various muscle groups. This may include leg lifts, arm curls, and core exercises using flotation devices or resistance bands.

6. **Cool Down and Stretching:** End each aquatic therapy session with a cool-down period to gradually lower heart rate and stretch tight muscles. Focus on gentle stretching exercises to improve flexibility and range of motion.

7. **Progression and Monitoring:** As you become more comfortable with aquatic therapy, gradually increase the intensity and duration of your

exercises. Monitor your progress and make adjustments to your program as needed to continue challenging yourself while avoiding overexertion.

Aquatic therapy offers numerous benefits for cardiovascular conditioning and overall rehabilitation in individuals recovering from stroke. By incorporating aquatic therapy into a comprehensive stroke recovery regimen under the guidance of a healthcare professional, individuals can improve cardiovascular fitness, muscle strength, balance, and coordination in a safe and supportive environment.

WALKING AND TREADMILL TRAINING

Walking and treadmill training are fundamental components of cardiovascular conditioning for individuals undergoing stroke recovery. These exercises are accessible, versatile, and effective for improving cardiovascular health, endurance, and mobility. Whether walking outdoors or using a treadmill indoors, these activities provide opportunities to increase heart rate, strengthen muscles, and enhance overall fitness levels. Here's how walking and treadmill training can benefit individuals recovering from stroke:

Benefits of Walking and Treadmill Training:

1. **Improved Cardiovascular Health:** Walking and treadmill training elevate heart rate, increase oxygen consumption, and improve circulation, leading to better cardiovascular health and reduced risk of heart disease.

2. **Enhanced Endurance:** Regular walking and treadmill training gradually increase aerobic capacity and stamina, allowing individuals to engage in daily activities with less fatigue and greater endurance.

3. **Muscle Strengthening:** Walking and treadmill training engage muscles throughout the body, including the legs, hips, core, and upper body, leading to improved strength and muscle tone.

4. **Improved Balance and Coordination:** Walking and treadmill training challenge balance and coordination, helping individuals improve stability and reduce the risk of falls.

5. **Weight Management:** Walking and treadmill training contribute to calorie expenditure and weight management, making them effective

components of a healthy lifestyle for individuals recovering from stroke.

6. **Enhanced Mood and Mental Health:** Walking and treadmill training release endorphins, which can improve mood, reduce stress, and enhance overall well-being.

Incorporating Walking and Treadmill Training into Stroke Recovery:

1. **Consultation with Healthcare Provider:** Before starting a walking or treadmill training program, individuals should consult with their healthcare provider or physical therapist to ensure it's safe and appropriate for their specific condition and needs.

2. **Assessment of Mobility and Fitness Levels:** Assess current mobility and fitness levels to determine the appropriate starting point for walking or treadmill training. Individuals may need to start with shorter durations or lower intensities and gradually progress as tolerated.

3. **Proper Footwear and Equipment:** Wear supportive, comfortable footwear with good traction to reduce the risk of slips and falls while

walking or using a treadmill. Ensure the treadmill is set up correctly with appropriate speed and incline settings.

4. **Start Slowly and Gradually Increase Intensity:** Begin with a comfortable pace and duration of walking or treadmill training, gradually increasing speed, duration, and incline as fitness improves. Aim for at least 20-30 minutes of moderate-intensity walking most days of the week.

5. **Use Handrails and Safety Features:** When using a treadmill, individuals should use handrails for support and safety, especially when starting or stopping the machine. Familiarize yourself with the emergency stop button and other safety features.

6. **Incorporate Variety:** To keep walking and treadmill training interesting and challenging, incorporate variety into the routine. This may include varying the speed, incline, and duration of treadmill sessions, as well as walking outdoors on different terrain.

7. **Monitor Progress:** Keep track of progress by recording distance, duration, and intensity of walking or treadmill sessions. Adjust the program

as needed to continue challenging yourself and meeting fitness goals.

Walking and treadmill training offer numerous benefits for cardiovascular conditioning and overall rehabilitation in individuals recovering from stroke. By incorporating these activities into a comprehensive stroke recovery regimen under the guidance of a healthcare professional, individuals can improve cardiovascular fitness, endurance, muscle strength, balance, and coordination, leading to improved overall health and quality of life.

CHAPTER 6

Flexibility Training

STRETCHING EXERCISES FOR FLEXIBILITY

Flexibility training is essential for individuals undergoing stroke recovery to improve range of motion, reduce muscle stiffness, and enhance overall mobility. Stretching exercises help lengthen muscles, tendons, and ligaments, increasing flexibility and reducing the risk of injury. Incorporating a regular stretching routine into a stroke recovery program can lead to improved functional abilities and better quality of life. Here are some effective stretching exercises for flexibility suitable for stroke recovery:

1. **Neck Stretches**:
   - Sit or stand with a tall posture, shoulders relaxed.
   - Slowly tilt the head to one side, bringing the ear towards the shoulder until a gentle stretch is felt along the side of the neck.

- Hold the stretch for 15-30 seconds, then return to the starting position and repeat on the opposite side.
- Perform 2-3 repetitions on each side, focusing on relaxing the neck muscles and avoiding any sudden or forceful movements.

2. **Shoulder Stretch**:
  - Stand tall with feet shoulder-width apart.
  - Reach one arm across the chest, using the opposite hand to gently press the arm closer to the body until a stretch is felt in the shoulder and upper back.
  - Hold the stretch for 15-30 seconds, then switch arms and repeat on the opposite side.
  - Perform 2-3 repetitions on each side, focusing on maintaining good posture and breathing deeply throughout the stretch.

3. **Chest Opener Stretch**:
  - Stand tall with feet hip-width apart and interlace fingers behind the back.
  - Gently straighten the arms and lift them away from the body, opening the chest and squeezing the shoulder blades together.
  - Hold the stretch for 15-30 seconds, focusing on keeping the chest lifted and the shoulders relaxed.

- Release the arms and repeat for 2-3 repetitions, breathing deeply and maintaining a steady pace.

4. **Trunk Rotation Stretch**:
   - Sit on the edge of a chair with feet flat on the floor and knees bent.
   - Place one hand on the outside of the opposite knee and gently rotate the torso towards that side, looking over the shoulder.
   - Hold the stretch for 15-30 seconds, feeling a gentle twist through the spine and torso.
   - Return to the starting position and repeat on the opposite side, performing 2-3 repetitions on each side.

5. **Hamstring Stretch**:
   - Sit on the floor with one leg extended straight in front and the other leg bent, foot flat on the floor.
   - Reach towards the extended leg, sliding the hands down the shin or towards the foot until a stretch is felt in the back of the thigh.
   - Hold the stretch for 15-30 seconds, breathing deeply and relaxing into the stretch.
   - Switch legs and repeat the stretch on the opposite side, performing 2-3 repetitions on each leg.

6. **Calf Stretch**:

   - Stand facing a wall with hands resting against the wall at shoulder height.

   - Step one foot back, keeping the heel flat on the floor and the knee straight.

   - Lean forward slightly, feeling a stretch in the calf of the back leg.

   - Hold the stretch for 15-30 seconds, then switch legs and repeat on the opposite side.

   - Perform 2-3 repetitions on each leg, focusing on keeping the heel firmly planted on the floor.

Perform these stretching exercises for flexibility 2-3 times per week, aiming for 1-3 sets of 15-30 seconds for each stretch. Focus on gentle, controlled movements and avoid bouncing or jerking during stretches. Incorporating flexibility training into a stroke recovery program can help individuals improve range of motion, reduce muscle tension, and enhance overall mobility and quality of life.

YOGA AND TAI CHI FOR STROKE RECOVERY

Yoga and Tai Chi are ancient practices that offer numerous physical and mental benefits, making them valuable components of flexibility training for individuals undergoing stroke recovery. Both Yoga and Tai Chi emphasize gentle, flowing movements, mindfulness, and breath control, making them accessible and suitable for people of all fitness levels, including those with mobility challenges. Incorporating these practices into a stroke recovery program can help improve flexibility, balance, strength, and overall well-being. Here's how Yoga and Tai Chi can benefit individuals recovering from stroke:

Benefits of Yoga and Tai Chi for Stroke Recovery:

1. **Improved Flexibility:** Both Yoga and Tai Chi incorporate stretching and gentle movements that help improve flexibility, range of motion, and joint mobility, which can be especially beneficial for individuals with muscle stiffness or spasticity after a stroke.

2. **Enhanced Balance and Coordination:** Yoga and Tai Chi involve various postures and movements that challenge balance and coordination, helping individuals improve stability and reduce the risk of falls.

3. **Stress Reduction:** The mindfulness and deep breathing techniques practiced in Yoga and Tai Chi

can help reduce stress, anxiety, and depression, promoting a sense of calm and relaxation.

4. **Increased Strength:** While Yoga and Tai Chi are primarily focused on flexibility and balance, they also involve engaging muscles throughout the body, leading to improved strength and muscle tone over time.

5. **Mind-Body Connection:** Both practices emphasize the connection between the mind and body, encouraging individuals to tune into their physical sensations, thoughts, and emotions, fostering greater self-awareness and resilience.

6. **Social Support:** Participating in group Yoga or Tai Chi classes provides opportunities for social interaction and support, which can be beneficial for overall well-being and motivation during stroke recovery.

Incorporating Yoga and Tai Chi into Stroke Recovery:

1. **Consultation with Healthcare Provider:** Before starting a Yoga or Tai Chi practice, individuals should consult with their healthcare

provider or physical therapist to ensure it's safe and appropriate for their specific condition and needs.

2. **Beginner-Friendly Classes:** Look for beginner-friendly Yoga or Tai Chi classes specifically designed for individuals with mobility challenges or disabilities. Many community centers, fitness studios, and rehabilitation facilities offer adapted classes tailored to various needs.

3. **Adaptations and Modifications:** Instructors can provide adaptations and modifications for individuals with limited mobility or specific physical limitations. Props such as chairs, bolsters, and straps can be used to support and modify poses as needed.

4. **Gradual Progression:** Start slowly and gradually increase the duration and intensity of your Yoga or Tai Chi practice as your strength, flexibility, and confidence improve. Listen to your body and honor your limitations, avoiding overexertion or pushing yourself too hard.

5. **Consistency and Practice:** Consistency is key to reaping the benefits of Yoga and Tai Chi for stroke recovery. Aim to practice regularly, whether

it's attending classes, following instructional videos, or practicing at home.

6. **Mindful Awareness:** Pay attention to your breath, body sensations, and thoughts during your practice, cultivating mindful awareness and presence in the moment. Use your breath to guide your movements and promote relaxation and ease.

7. **Enjoyment and Exploration:** Approach Yoga and Tai Chi with an open mind and a spirit of curiosity and exploration. Experiment with different styles, teachers, and practices to find what resonates best with you and brings you joy and fulfillment.

By incorporating Yoga and Tai Chi into a comprehensive stroke recovery program, individuals can reap the numerous physical, mental, and emotional benefits of these ancient practices. With guidance from healthcare professionals and instructors, Yoga and Tai Chi can help individuals improve flexibility, balance, strength, and overall well-being, supporting their journey towards recovery and optimal health.

CHAPTER 7

Functional Training

ACTIVITIES OF DAILY LIVING (ADL) TRAINING

Activities of Daily Living (ADL) training is a crucial component of functional training for individuals undergoing stroke recovery. ADLs are routine tasks that people perform as part of their daily lives, such as bathing, dressing, grooming, eating, and mobility. Stroke survivors often experience difficulties with these activities due to physical impairments, weakness, or cognitive challenges. ADL training focuses on regaining independence and improving functional abilities to perform these tasks safely and efficiently. Here's how ADL training can benefit stroke recovery:

Benefits of ADL Training:

1. **Promotes Independence:** ADL training helps stroke survivors regain independence in performing essential daily tasks, enhancing their quality of life and sense of self-esteem and autonomy.

2. **Improves Functional Abilities:** By practicing ADLs, individuals can improve physical strength, coordination, balance, and cognitive skills necessary for performing everyday activities.

3. **Enhances Confidence:** Successfully completing ADLs reinforces confidence and self-efficacy, empowering stroke survivors to overcome challenges and achieve greater independence.

4. **Facilitates Rehabilitation:** ADL training is an integral part of stroke rehabilitation, providing opportunities for practice, repetition, and skill refinement in real-life contexts.

5. **Supports Goal-Oriented Therapy:** ADL training allows therapists to set functional goals tailored to each individual's needs and priorities, providing a meaningful framework for rehabilitation.

6. **Addresses Safety Concerns:** Learning proper techniques and strategies for ADLs reduces the risk of accidents, falls, and injuries during daily activities, promoting a safer home environment.

Incorporating ADL Training into Stroke Recovery:

1. **Assessment of Functional Abilities:** Begin by assessing the individual's current abilities and challenges related to ADLs, considering physical, cognitive, and environmental factors. Identify specific tasks that require improvement or modification.

2. **Task Analysis:** Break down each ADL task into smaller, manageable steps, considering the physical, cognitive, and environmental demands involved. Identify any barriers or obstacles that may hinder task performance.

3. **Skill Building:** Use a combination of hands-on instruction, demonstration, verbal cues, and visual aids to teach and reinforce proper techniques for performing ADLs. Provide opportunities for practice and repetition to build skills and confidence.

4. **Adaptations and Modifications:** Modify ADL tasks or environments as needed to accommodate individual abilities and limitations. Use adaptive equipment, assistive devices, or environmental

modifications to facilitate task performance and promote independence.

5. **Progressive Training:** Gradually increase the complexity, difficulty, or independence level of ADL tasks as the individual's abilities improve. Set realistic goals and celebrate achievements along the way to maintain motivation and momentum.

6. **Functional Context:** Incorporate ADL training into real-life contexts and environments, such as the home or community setting, to enhance relevance and transferability of skills. Practice tasks in settings where they will be performed regularly.

7. **Multidisciplinary Collaboration:** Coordinate ADL training efforts with other members of the rehabilitation team, including physical therapists, occupational therapists, speech therapists, and caregivers, to ensure a comprehensive and holistic approach to stroke recovery.

Examples of ADL training activities may include:

- Dressing practice, including putting on and taking off clothing, fastening buttons, and tying shoelaces.
- Bathing and grooming tasks, such as washing, combing hair, brushing teeth, and shaving.

- Meal preparation and eating, including cooking, cutting food, using utensils, and swallowing safely.
- Mobility and transfers, such as getting in and out of bed, standing up from a chair, and walking safely with or without assistive devices.

By incorporating ADL training into a comprehensive stroke recovery program, individuals can regain independence, improve functional abilities, and enhance their overall quality of life. With tailored instruction, support, and practice, stroke survivors can overcome challenges and achieve greater autonomy in performing activities of daily living.

OCCUPATIONAL THERAPY EXERCISES

Occupational therapy (OT) exercises play a vital role in functional training for individuals undergoing stroke recovery. Occupational therapists focus on improving a person's ability to perform daily activities and tasks, such as self-care, work-related tasks, and leisure activities, to promote independence and enhance quality of life. OT exercises are designed to address specific functional goals and challenges faced by stroke survivors, helping them regain skills and adapt to any physical or cognitive impairments. Here's how occupational therapy exercises can benefit stroke recovery:

Benefits of Occupational Therapy Exercises:

1. **Task-Specific Training:** Occupational therapy exercises are tailored to address the individual's specific needs and functional goals, focusing on tasks that are meaningful and relevant to their daily life.

2. **Improves Functional Independence:** By targeting activities of daily living (ADLs) and instrumental activities of daily living (IADLs), occupational therapy exercises help stroke survivors regain independence in essential tasks such as dressing, grooming, cooking, and managing finances.

3. **Enhances Motor Skills:** OT exercises focus on improving motor skills, coordination, and fine motor control needed for tasks such as grasping objects, manipulating utensils, and using tools or adaptive devices.

4. **Addresses Cognitive Challenges:** Occupational therapists incorporate cognitive rehabilitation techniques into exercises to address

memory, attention, problem-solving, and executive functioning deficits commonly experienced after a stroke.

5. **Promotes Adaptation and Compensation:** OT exercises teach stroke survivors strategies to adapt to any physical or cognitive impairments, such as using assistive devices, modifying task techniques, or implementing memory aids, to facilitate task performance and maximize independence.

6. **Prevents Secondary Complications:** Occupational therapy exercises aim to prevent secondary complications such as muscle weakness, contractures, and joint stiffness by promoting movement, mobility, and active engagement in daily activities.

Examples of Occupational Therapy Exercises:

1. **Fine Motor Exercises:**
   - Finger and hand exercises using therapy putty, grip strengthening devices, or hand therapy balls to improve dexterity and coordination.
   - Pegboard activities to practice fine motor control, precision, and manipulation skills.

- Writing or drawing exercises to improve handwriting or artistic abilities, focusing on pencil grasp, control, and letter formation.

2. **Activities of Daily Living (ADL) Training:**
    - Dressing practice, including putting on and taking off clothing, fastening buttons, zipping zippers, and tying shoelaces.
    - Grooming tasks such as brushing hair, shaving, applying makeup, and brushing teeth to promote self-care independence.
    - Meal preparation and cooking activities, including chopping vegetables, stirring ingredients, and using kitchen utensils to enhance cooking skills and safety awareness.

3. **Balance and Coordination Exercises:**
    - Standing balance activities such as weight shifting, reaching, and transferring weight between legs to improve stability and reduce the risk of falls.
    - Coordination drills involving bilateral movements, reaching, grasping, and manipulating objects to enhance coordination and motor planning.

4. **Cognitive Rehabilitation Tasks:**
    - Memory games and exercises to improve short-term memory, attention, and recall.

- Problem-solving activities such as puzzles, sequencing tasks, and strategy games to enhance cognitive flexibility and executive functioning skills.

- Safety awareness and decision-making exercises to promote independence and self-management skills in daily activities.

5. **Environmental Modification and Assistive Device Training:**

- Home assessment and modification to identify barriers and make adaptations to the environment to enhance safety and accessibility.

- Training in the use of assistive devices such as adaptive equipment, mobility aids, or electronic devices to compensate for functional limitations and promote independence.

Occupational therapy exercises are typically prescribed based on individual needs, goals, and functional abilities. Occupational therapists work closely with stroke survivors to develop personalized treatment plans and provide ongoing support, guidance, and encouragement throughout the rehabilitation process. By incorporating occupational therapy exercises into a comprehensive stroke recovery program, individuals can regain skills, adapt to challenges, and achieve greater independence and participation in daily life activities.

CHAPTER 8

TIPS FOR SAFE AND EFFECTIVE WORKOUTS

MONITORING INTENSITY LEVELS

Monitoring intensity levels during workouts is crucial for ensuring safety and effectiveness, especially for individuals undergoing stroke recovery. Understanding and controlling exercise intensity helps prevent overexertion, minimize the risk of injury, and optimize the benefits of physical activity. Here are some tips for monitoring intensity levels during workouts:

1. **Know Your Baseline:** Before starting any exercise program, it's essential to know your baseline fitness level and any physical limitations or medical conditions. Consult with a healthcare professional or physical therapist to assess your current fitness status and establish appropriate exercise goals.

2. **Use Perceived Exertion:** Pay attention to how your body feels during exercise and use the Borg Rating of Perceived Exertion (RPE) scale to gauge

intensity. This subjective scale ranges from 6 to 20, with 6 representing no exertion and 20 representing maximal exertion. Aim to maintain an RPE of around 11-14 during moderate-intensity exercise and 15-17 during vigorous-intensity exercise.

3. **Monitor Heart Rate:** Monitoring heart rate can provide objective feedback on exercise intensity. Use a heart rate monitor or take your pulse manually to track heart rate during exercise. Aim to stay within your target heart rate zone based on your age and fitness level, typically around 50-85% of your maximum heart rate.

4. **Use Talk Test:** The talk test is a simple way to gauge exercise intensity based on your ability to speak comfortably during exercise. During moderate-intensity exercise, you should be able to carry on a conversation without difficulty. If you're unable to speak comfortably due to breathlessness, the intensity may be too high.

5. **Watch for Signs of Overexertion:** Be aware of warning signs of overexertion, such as dizziness, lightheadedness, shortness of breath, chest pain, nausea, or excessive fatigue. If you experience any of these symptoms, stop exercising immediately

and rest. Seek medical attention if symptoms persist or worsen.

6. **Gradually Increase Intensity:** Start with low to moderate-intensity exercises and gradually increase intensity over time as fitness improves. Avoid sudden spikes in intensity or volume, as this can increase the risk of injury or setbacks in recovery.

7. **Listen to Your Body:** Pay attention to your body's signals and adjust exercise intensity accordingly. If you're feeling tired or fatigued, take a break or reduce the intensity of your workout. It's important to strike a balance between challenging yourself and avoiding excessive strain.

8. **Stay Hydrated:** Drink plenty of water before, during, and after exercise to maintain hydration levels, especially during intense or prolonged workouts. Dehydration can negatively impact exercise performance and increase the risk of heat-related illnesses.

9. **Modify Exercises as Needed:** If you have physical limitations or mobility challenges, modify exercises to suit your abilities. Focus on exercises that are safe and comfortable for your body, and

don't hesitate to ask for guidance from a qualified fitness professional or physical therapist.

10. **Track Progress:** Keep a workout journal or use a fitness app to track your exercise sessions, including duration, intensity, and any relevant notes. Monitoring progress can help you stay motivated and identify areas for improvement.

By monitoring intensity levels during workouts and adjusting accordingly, individuals undergoing stroke recovery can ensure safe and effective exercise participation, leading to improved fitness, function, and overall well-being. Always consult with a healthcare professional before starting a new exercise program, especially if you have underlying health conditions or concerns.

USING ASSISTIVE DEVICES IF NECESSARY
For individuals undergoing stroke recovery or with mobility challenges, using assistive devices during workouts can enhance safety, accessibility, and effectiveness. Assistive devices provide support, stability, and assistance with movement, allowing individuals to participate in physical activity with confidence and independence. Here are some tips for using assistive devices safely and effectively during workouts:

1. **Choose the Right Device:** Select an assistive device that meets your specific needs and abilities. Common assistive devices for exercise include canes, walkers, crutches, wheelchairs, and mobility scooters. Consider factors such as stability, maneuverability, weight capacity, and adjustability when choosing a device.

2. **Proper Fit and Adjustment:** Ensure that the assistive device is properly fitted and adjusted to your height, weight, and body proportions. Seek guidance from a healthcare professional or physical therapist to ensure correct sizing and positioning of the device for optimal support and comfort.

3. **Practice Proper Technique:** Learn and practice proper techniques for using the assistive device, including how to stand, walk, sit, and transfer safely. Use good posture, engage core muscles, and distribute weight evenly to minimize strain on joints and muscles.

4. **Gradual Progression:** Start slowly and gradually increase the intensity and duration of exercise while using the assistive device. Allow time to adapt to the device and build strength, endurance, and confidence over time. Avoid overexertion or pushing beyond your limits.

5. **Use Stability Aids:** If balance is a concern, consider using stability aids such as handrails, grab bars, or wall-mounted supports during exercise. These aids provide additional stability and safety when performing standing exercises or activities that require balance.

6. **Adapt Exercises as Needed:** Modify exercises to accommodate the use of assistive devices and any physical limitations. Focus on exercises that are safe, comfortable, and appropriate for your abilities. Use props, chairs, or benches for support and stability as needed.

7. **Seek Professional Guidance:** Consult with a physical therapist, occupational therapist, or certified fitness professional for guidance on using assistive devices during workouts. They can provide personalized recommendations, exercises, and techniques to maximize safety and effectiveness.

8. **Monitor Device Condition:** Regularly inspect the assistive device for signs of wear, damage, or malfunction. Replace worn-out parts or components as needed to ensure the device remains safe and functional during exercise.

9. **Stay Hydrated:** Drink water regularly before, during, and after exercise to stay hydrated, especially when using assistive devices that may increase exertion or effort. Dehydration can affect performance and increase the risk of fatigue or overheating.

10. **Listen to Your Body:** Pay attention to your body's signals and adjust exercise intensity or technique as needed. If you experience discomfort, pain, or fatigue, stop exercising and rest. Listen to your body's cues and avoid pushing through pain or discomfort.

Using assistive devices during workouts can empower individuals with mobility challenges to participate in physical activity safely and effectively. By choosing the right device, practicing proper technique, gradually progressing, and seeking professional guidance, individuals can enhance their exercise experience and improve overall fitness, function, and well-being.

PREVENTING OVEREXERTION AND INJURY

Preventing overexertion and injury during workouts is essential for individuals undergoing stroke recovery or those with mobility challenges.

Overexertion can lead to fatigue, muscle strain, joint pain, and even serious injuries, hindering progress and impeding recovery. By following these tips, individuals can reduce the risk of overexertion and injury during exercise:

1. **Start Slowly and Gradually:** Begin with low-intensity exercises and gradually increase the duration, intensity, and complexity of workouts over time. Allow your body to adapt to the demands of exercise and avoid sudden spikes in activity that may lead to overexertion.

2. **Warm-Up Properly:** Always start with a proper warm-up to prepare your body for exercise. Incorporate dynamic movements such as arm swings, leg swings, and marching in place to increase blood flow, loosen muscles, and improve flexibility.

3. **Listen to Your Body:** Pay attention to how your body feels during exercise and respect its limitations. If you experience pain, discomfort, dizziness, or unusual fatigue, stop exercising immediately and rest. Pushing through pain or discomfort can lead to injury.

4. **Stay Hydrated:** Drink water before, during, and after exercise to maintain hydration levels and prevent dehydration. Dehydration can impair performance, increase fatigue, and raise the risk of overheating or heat-related illnesses.

5. **Use Proper Form:** Maintain proper form and technique during exercises to avoid placing excessive stress on joints, muscles, and ligaments. Focus on controlled movements, alignment, and posture to minimize the risk of injury.

6. **Incorporate Rest and Recovery:** Allow adequate time for rest and recovery between workouts to prevent overtraining and promote muscle repair and growth. Aim for at least one or two days of rest each week, and listen to your body's signals for fatigue and recovery needs.

7. **Balance Cardiovascular and Strength Training:** Incorporate a mix of cardiovascular (e.g., walking, cycling) and strength training (e.g., resistance exercises) into your workout routine. Balancing different types of exercise helps prevent overuse injuries and promotes overall fitness and function.

8. **Use Assistive Devices if Necessary:** If you have mobility challenges or limitations, use assistive devices such as canes, walkers, or mobility aids to provide support and stability during exercise. Choose devices that are appropriate for your needs and properly fitted to your body.

9. **Avoid Overdoing It:** Pace yourself during workouts and avoid pushing beyond your limits. Set realistic goals and progress gradually over time. Remember that consistency and moderation are key to long-term success and injury prevention.

10. **Cool Down Properly:** Finish each workout with a proper cool down to help your body return to a resting state gradually. Incorporate static stretches for major muscle groups to improve flexibility and reduce muscle soreness.

11. **Seek Professional Guidance:** Consult with a healthcare professional, physical therapist, or certified fitness trainer for personalized guidance and exercise recommendations. They can help you design a safe and effective workout program tailored to your specific needs and abilities.

By following these tips, individuals can reduce the risk of overexertion and injury during workouts, promoting safe and effective exercise participation and supporting overall health and well-being. Remember to prioritize safety, listen to your body, and seek professional guidance as needed to maximize the benefits of physical activity.

CHAPTER 9

Sample Workout Routines

BEGINNER'S ROUTINE

For individuals new to exercise or those beginning their journey in stroke recovery, a beginner's workout routine provides a gentle introduction to physical activity while building strength, flexibility, and endurance gradually. This sample workout routine focuses on low-impact exercises that are safe and accessible for beginners. Always consult with a healthcare professional or physical therapist before starting any new exercise program, especially if you have underlying health conditions or concerns.

Warm-Up:
- Duration: 5-10 minutes
- Activities:
    - Arm circles: 10-15 repetitions forward and backward
  - Leg swings: 10-15 swings for each leg
  - Marching in place: 1-2 minutes
  - Gentle neck stretches: Hold for 15-20 seconds on each side

   - Shoulder rolls: 10-15 repetitions forward and backward

Cardiovascular Exercise:
- Duration: 10-15 minutes
- Activities:
   - Walking: Start with a brisk walk for 5-10 minutes, gradually increasing duration over time.
   - Stationary cycling: Pedal at a comfortable pace on a stationary bike for 10-15 minutes.
   - Water aerobics: Participate in a water aerobics class or perform gentle movements in a swimming pool for cardiovascular conditioning.

Strength Training:
- Duration: 10-15 minutes
- Exercises:
  - Bodyweight squats: 2 sets of 8-12 repetitions
  - Wall push-ups: 2 sets of 8-12 repetitions
  - Seated leg lifts: 2 sets of 8-12 repetitions for each leg
   - Bicep curls with light dumbbells or resistance bands: 2 sets of 8-12 repetitions
   - Seated or standing rows with resistance bands: 2 sets of 8-12 repetitions

Flexibility and Stretching:
- Duration: 5-10 minutes

- Exercises:
    - Neck stretches: Hold each stretch for 15-20 seconds, repeating on each side.
    - Shoulder stretches: Gently stretch each shoulder by crossing the arm across the body and holding for 15-20 seconds.
    - Hamstring stretches: Sit on the floor with one leg extended and gently reach towards the toes, holding for 15-20 seconds on each leg.
    - Quadriceps stretches: Stand or lie on your side, gently pulling one foot towards the glutes, holding for 15-20 seconds on each leg.
    - Calf stretches: Stand facing a wall with one foot behind the other, gently leaning forward to stretch the calf muscle, holding for 15-20 seconds on each leg.

Cool Down:
- Duration: 5-10 minutes
- Activities:
    - Slow walking or marching in place for 3-5 minutes to gradually lower heart rate.
    - Gentle stretching for major muscle groups, holding each stretch for 15-20 seconds.
    - Deep breathing exercises or relaxation techniques to promote a sense of calm and relaxation.

Guidelines:
- Start with shorter durations and lower intensities, gradually increasing as tolerated.
- Perform each exercise with proper form and technique to avoid injury.
- Listen to your body and rest as needed. If you experience pain or discomfort, stop exercising and consult with a healthcare professional.
- Stay hydrated by drinking water before, during, and after exercise.
- Aim to perform this beginner's workout routine 2-3 times per week, gradually progressing as fitness improves.

This beginner's workout routine provides a well-rounded approach to exercise, incorporating cardiovascular, strength, flexibility, and relaxation components. As individuals become more comfortable with the exercises, they can gradually increase the duration, intensity, and complexity of their workouts to continue challenging themselves and promoting progress in stroke recovery.

INTERMEDIATE ROUTINE
For individuals who have progressed beyond the beginner level in their stroke recovery journey or have been exercising regularly and want to challenge themselves further, an intermediate

workout routine provides a more intensive and varied approach to fitness. This sample intermediate routine includes a combination of cardiovascular, strength, flexibility, and balance exercises to continue improving overall health and functional abilities. As always, consult with a healthcare professional or physical therapist before starting any new exercise program, especially if you have underlying health conditions or concerns.

Warm-Up:
- Duration: 5-10 minutes
- Activities:
   - Arm circles: 10-15 repetitions forward and backward
  - Leg swings: 10-15 swings for each leg
  - Marching in place with high knees: 1-2 minutes
  - Neck rotations: Slowly rotate the neck in each direction, 5-10 repetitions
   - Shoulder rolls: 10-15 repetitions forward and backward

Cardiovascular Exercise:
- Duration: 20-30 minutes
- Activities:
   - Brisk walking or jogging: 20-30 minutes at a moderate to vigorous intensity

- Cycling: 20-30 minutes on a stationary bike or outdoor bike at a challenging pace

- Swimming: Perform laps or water aerobics for 20-30 minutes to elevate heart rate and improve cardiovascular fitness

Strength Training:
- Duration: 20-30 minutes
- Exercises:
  - Squats: 3 sets of 10-12 repetitions with or without added resistance (dumbbells, resistance bands)
  - Lunges: 3 sets of 10-12 repetitions for each leg
  - Push-ups: 3 sets of 8-10 repetitions (modified or full push-ups depending on ability)
  - Seated or standing rows: 3 sets of 10-12 repetitions with resistance bands or cable machine
  - Dumbbell or kettlebell swings: 3 sets of 10-12 repetitions to improve power and strength in the lower body and core

Flexibility and Stretching:
- Duration: 10-15 minutes
- Exercises:
  - Dynamic stretches: Perform dynamic movements such as leg swings, arm circles, and trunk rotations to improve flexibility and range of motion.
  - Static stretches: Hold stretches for major muscle groups (hamstrings, quadriceps, calves, chest,

shoulders) for 15-30 seconds each, repeating 2-3 times.

Balance and Stability Training:
- Duration: 10-15 minutes
- Activities:
  - Single-leg balance: Stand on one leg for 30-60 seconds, alternating legs.
  - Balance exercises on unstable surfaces (BOSU ball, balance board): Perform exercises such as squats, lunges, and arm reaches to challenge balance and stability.
  - Tai Chi or yoga poses: Incorporate balance-focused poses such as tree pose, warrior III, or eagle pose to improve balance and coordination.

Cool Down:
- Duration: 5-10 minutes
- Activities:
  - Slow walking or marching in place for 3-5 minutes to gradually lower heart rate.
  - Gentle stretching for major muscle groups, holding each stretch for 15-30 seconds.
  - Deep breathing exercises or relaxation techniques to promote relaxation and recovery.

Guidelines:
- Gradually increase the intensity, duration, and complexity of exercises as fitness improves.
- Maintain proper form and technique during strength training exercises to avoid injury.
- Allow adequate rest and recovery between workout sessions to prevent overtraining.
- Stay hydrated by drinking water before, during, and after exercise.
- Listen to your body and adjust exercise intensity or technique as needed. If you experience pain or discomfort, stop exercising and consult with a healthcare professional.

This intermediate workout routine provides a balanced and challenging approach to exercise, incorporating a variety of activities to improve cardiovascular fitness, strength, flexibility, balance, and stability. As individuals progress in their stroke recovery or fitness journey, they can continue to adjust and modify their workouts to meet their evolving needs and goals.

ADVANCED ROUTINE
For individuals who have achieved a high level of fitness and functional ability in their stroke recovery journey or have been consistently exercising at an intermediate level and are ready for

further challenge, an advanced workout routine offers a more demanding and comprehensive approach to fitness. This sample advanced routine includes a combination of cardiovascular, strength, flexibility, balance, and functional exercises to promote peak physical performance and functional independence. As always, consult with a healthcare professional or physical therapist before starting any new exercise program, especially if you have underlying health conditions or concerns.

Warm-Up:
- Duration: 10-15 minutes
- Activities:

    - Dynamic stretching: Perform dynamic movements such as leg swings, arm circles, high knees, and butt kicks to loosen muscles and increase range of motion.

  - Joint mobility exercises: Include movements that target all major joints (shoulders, hips, knees, ankles) to prepare the body for more intense exercise.

Cardiovascular Exercise:
- Duration: 30-45 minutes
- Activities:

- Running or jogging: Incorporate intervals of varying speeds and intensities to challenge cardiovascular fitness and improve endurance.

- High-intensity interval training (HIIT): Alternate between periods of high-intensity exercise (e.g., sprinting, jumping jacks, burpees) and active recovery (e.g., walking, jogging) for maximum cardiovascular benefits.

- Cycling: Perform hill intervals or tempo rides on a stationary bike or outdoor bike to increase heart rate and improve aerobic capacity.

Strength Training:
- Duration: 30-45 minutes
- Exercises:

- Compound exercises: Incorporate multi-joint movements such as squats, deadlifts, lunges, push-ups, and pull-ups to engage multiple muscle groups simultaneously.

- Olympic lifts: Include power cleans, snatches, and overhead presses to improve explosive strength, power, and coordination.

- Plyometric exercises: Perform explosive movements such as box jumps, jump squats, and medicine ball throws to develop power and agility.

Flexibility and Mobility Work:
- Duration: 15-20 minutes

- Activities:
  - Dynamic stretches: Perform dynamic movements such as leg swings, arm circles, lunges with twists, and cat-cow stretches to improve flexibility and mobility.
  - Foam rolling: Use a foam roller to release tension in muscles and fascia, focusing on areas of tightness and discomfort.

Balance and Stability Training:
- Duration: 15-20 minutes
- Activities:
  - Single-leg balance exercises: Challenge balance and stability by performing single-leg squats, reaches, and hops.
  - Unstable surface training: Use balance boards, stability balls, or BOSU balls to perform exercises such as squats, lunges, and planks to enhance proprioception and core stability.

Functional Exercises:
- Duration: 20-30 minutes
- Activities:
  - Functional movement patterns: Incorporate exercises that mimic everyday movements such as bending, lifting, pushing, and pulling to improve overall functional capacity.

- Agility drills: Perform ladder drills, cone drills, or agility ladder exercises to enhance agility, coordination, and quickness.

Cool Down and Recovery:
- Duration: 10-15 minutes
- Activities:
    - Static stretching: Hold stretches for major muscle groups (hamstrings, quadriceps, calves, chest, shoulders) for 20-30 seconds each to improve flexibility and reduce muscle soreness.
    - Foam rolling: Use a foam roller to massage muscles and promote recovery, focusing on areas of tightness and discomfort.
    - Deep breathing exercises or meditation: Practice relaxation techniques to promote mental and physical relaxation and aid in recovery.

Guidelines:
- Gradually progress intensity, duration, and complexity of exercises over time to avoid overtraining and injury.
- Listen to your body and adjust exercise intensity or technique as needed. If you experience pain or discomfort, stop exercising and consult with a healthcare professional.

- Incorporate variety and challenge into your workouts to prevent plateaus and promote continuous improvement.
- Stay hydrated by drinking water before, during, and after exercise, especially during intense workouts.
- Prioritize adequate rest and recovery between workout sessions to allow muscles to repair and grow.
- Focus on proper form and technique during exercises to maximize effectiveness and reduce the risk of injury.

This advanced workout routine is designed to push individuals to their limits and optimize physical performance while promoting functional independence and overall well-being. As with any exercise program, it's important to listen to your body, respect your limits, and seek professional guidance as needed to ensure safe and effective training.

CHAPTER 10

TRACKING PROGRESS AND ADJUSTMENTS

KEEPING A WORKOUT JOURNAL

Keeping a workout journal is a valuable tool for individuals undergoing stroke recovery or engaging in any fitness program. A workout journal helps track progress, monitor performance, and make necessary adjustments to optimize training and achieve goals effectively. Whether handwritten in a notebook or digitally using a fitness app, a workout journal provides a record of workouts, exercises, sets, reps, intensity, and other relevant metrics. Here's how keeping a workout journal can benefit stroke recovery and fitness progress:

Benefits of Keeping a Workout Journal:

1. **Progress Tracking:** A workout journal allows individuals to track their progress over time, including improvements in strength, endurance, flexibility, and overall fitness. Recording workouts and performance metrics provides tangible

evidence of progress and motivates continued effort and commitment.

2. **Identifying Patterns and Trends:** By documenting workouts and related factors such as sleep, nutrition, and stress levels, individuals can identify patterns and trends that impact performance and recovery. This information helps make informed decisions about training strategies, recovery practices, and lifestyle adjustments.

3. **Setting and Achieving Goals:** A workout journal helps individuals set specific, measurable, achievable, relevant, and time-bound (SMART) goals for their stroke recovery or fitness journey. Tracking progress towards these goals provides clarity, focus, and motivation to stay on track and achieve success.

4. **Monitoring Performance:** Recording workout details such as sets, reps, weights, and rest periods helps individuals monitor performance and identify areas for improvement. Tracking performance metrics allows for progressive overload, ensuring that workouts remain challenging and effective for continued progress.

5. **Accountability and Compliance:** Keeping a workout journal promotes accountability and adherence to the exercise program. The act of recording workouts encourages consistency, discipline, and commitment to regular exercise, reducing the likelihood of missed workouts or deviations from the plan.

6. **Individualized Programming:** A workout journal provides valuable data for designing and adjusting individualized exercise programs based on specific needs, goals, and preferences. By reviewing past workouts and progress, individuals can tailor their training to address strengths, weaknesses, and areas for improvement.

7. **Injury Prevention:** Monitoring workload and training volume in a workout journal helps prevent overtraining and reduce the risk of injury. Recognizing signs of fatigue, overuse, or imbalance allows for appropriate adjustments to training intensity, frequency, and recovery strategies.

Tips for Keeping a Workout Journal:

1. **Record Key Details:** Include essential information such as date, time, duration, type of workout, exercises performed, sets, reps, weights,

intensity, and perceived exertion (e.g., using the Borg RPE scale).

2. **Be Consistent:** Make it a habit to record workouts immediately after completion while details are fresh in your mind. Consistency in journaling ensures accurate tracking and allows for meaningful analysis of progress.

3. **Use Descriptive Notes:** Include descriptive notes or comments about each workout, such as how you felt, any modifications made, challenges encountered, and areas of improvement. This qualitative feedback provides context and insights into performance and progress.

4. **Review and Reflect:** Regularly review and reflect on your workout journal to assess progress, identify trends, and set new goals. Use this information to adjust training variables, modify workout plans, and plan future workouts accordingly.

5. **Celebrate Achievements:** Celebrate milestones, achievements, and progress milestones recorded in your workout journal. Recognizing progress boosts motivation, confidence, and commitment to continued effort and improvement.

6. **Stay Flexible:** Be open to making adjustments to your workout plan based on feedback from your workout journal, changes in goals, or fluctuations in health and fitness levels. Adaptability is key to long-term success and sustainability in your exercise program.

By keeping a workout journal, individuals can track progress, monitor performance, and make informed decisions to optimize their stroke recovery or fitness journey. Whether you're a beginner or advanced exerciser, maintaining a detailed record of your workouts provides valuable insights and accountability, supporting continued progress and success.

MODIFYING ROUTINES AS ABILITIES IMPROVE

In the journey of stroke recovery or any fitness program, adapting routines to reflect improvements in abilities is crucial for sustained progress and overall well-being. As individuals regain strength, mobility, and functionality, it's essential to adjust workout routines accordingly to ensure continued challenge and growth. Here's a comprehensive guide on how to track progress and make necessary adjustments to routines as abilities improve:

1. Regular Assessments:

- **Functional Evaluations:** Conduct periodic assessments to evaluate functional abilities such as mobility, strength, balance, and coordination. These assessments can help gauge progress and identify areas needing improvement.

- **Performance Metrics:** Keep track of performance metrics such as weights lifted, repetitions completed, distances walked or run, and exercise duration. Comparing current data to initial baseline measurements provides insight into progress.

- **Subjective Feedback:** Pay attention to how you feel during and after workouts. Notice any improvements in energy levels, reduced fatigue, enhanced mood, and increased confidence in performing daily activities. These subjective indicators reflect progress.

2. Signs of Improvement:

- **Increased Strength:** Notice improvements in strength by lifting heavier weights, completing more repetitions, or performing exercises with better form and control.

- **Enhanced Mobility:** Experience greater ease and range of motion in daily activities, along with reduced stiffness and discomfort in joints.

- **Improved Balance and Coordination:** Feel more stable and confident in maintaining balance during static and dynamic activities. Notice smoother and more controlled movements with less reliance on support or assistive devices.

- **Enhanced Endurance:** Notice increased stamina and reduced fatigue during cardiovascular activities, allowing for longer durations or higher intensities of exercise.

3. Modifying Routines:

- **Progressive Overload:** Gradually increase the intensity, duration, or difficulty of exercises to continue challenging your body and stimulating adaptation. Increase resistance, repetitions, or sets as abilities improve.

- **Advanced Exercise Variations:** Progress to more challenging variations or progressions of exercises to target muscles in new ways. For instance, advance from basic lunges to reverse lunges or add instability to exercises using balance boards or stability balls.

   - **Increased Training Volume:** Consider adding more sets, reps, or exercises to your routine as your capacity improves. This can help further develop strength, endurance, and muscle definition.

   - **Specialized Training:** Introduce specialized training techniques or modalities that align with your goals and interests. Incorporate interval training, plyometrics, or functional movements to enhance performance and functional capacity.

4. Monitoring and Feedback:

   - **Regular Reflection:** Schedule regular check-ins to reflect on progress and reassess goals. Modify routines based on feedback from assessments and subjective observations.

   - **Listening to Your Body:** Pay attention to signals from your body during workouts. Adjust intensity, volume, or exercise selection based on fatigue, discomfort, or any signs of overexertion.

   - **Professional Guidance:** Seek input from healthcare professionals, physical therapists, or certified trainers to ensure adjustments align with your individual needs and goals. They can provide personalized recommendations and support as you progress.

5. Celebrating Milestones:

   - **Acknowledge Achievements:** Celebrate milestones and accomplishments along the way. Recognizing progress boosts motivation and reinforces the importance of ongoing effort and dedication.

By tracking progress and making adjustments to routines as abilities improve, individuals can maintain momentum and continue progressing in their stroke recovery or fitness journey. Embrace the journey of growth and adaptation, and remember to listen to your body's cues to ensure safe and effective progress.

CHAPTER 11

ADDITIONAL RESOURCES

ONLINE COMMUNITIES AND SUPPORT GROUPS

Online communities and support groups play a vital role in providing encouragement, information, and camaraderie for individuals undergoing stroke recovery or participating in fitness programs. These virtual platforms offer a sense of belonging, connection, and empowerment, allowing members to share experiences, ask questions, and receive support from peers facing similar challenges. Here's how online communities and support groups can benefit individuals in their stroke recovery or fitness journey:

1. Peer Support:
   - Connect with individuals who understand the unique challenges and experiences associated with stroke recovery or fitness endeavors.
   - Share personal stories, successes, and struggles in a non-judgmental and supportive environment.

- Receive encouragement, empathy, and motivation from fellow members who are on similar paths.

2. Information and Resources:
- Access a wealth of information, resources, and educational materials related to stroke recovery, exercise physiology, nutrition, and wellness.
- Learn about new research, treatment options, and evidence-based practices from experts and fellow community members.
- Gain insights into effective strategies, techniques, and tools for optimizing recovery and achieving fitness goals.

3. Practical Advice and Tips:
- Receive practical advice, tips, and recommendations from experienced members and professionals on managing symptoms, overcoming challenges, and staying motivated.
- Learn about adaptive equipment, assistive devices, and modifications that can facilitate exercise participation and daily living activities.
- Share strategies for incorporating exercise into daily routines, setting realistic goals, and maintaining consistency in workouts.

4. Emotional Support and Empowerment:
- Find a safe space to express emotions, fears, and uncertainties about stroke recovery or fitness journey without fear of judgment.
- Receive encouragement, validation, and empowerment from peers and moderators to navigate obstacles and setbacks with resilience and optimism.
- Build confidence, self-esteem, and a sense of empowerment by celebrating achievements and milestones, no matter how small.

5. Accountability and Motivation:
- Set goals, track progress, and celebrate achievements within the community to stay accountable and motivated.
- Participate in challenges, virtual events, and group activities to foster a sense of camaraderie and friendly competition.
- Draw inspiration from success stories, transformations, and shared experiences of fellow members to stay focused and committed to your recovery or fitness journey.

6. Accessible Anytime, Anywhere:
- Benefit from the convenience and flexibility of accessing support and information anytime,

anywhere, from the comfort of your home or on the go.

- Engage in discussions, ask questions, and seek support at your own pace, without time constraints or geographical limitations.

7. Professional Guidance and Expert Advice:
- Interact with healthcare professionals, therapists, trainers, and experts who may participate or provide guidance within the community.

- Seek answers to specific questions, receive personalized recommendations, and clarify doubts regarding exercise programs, rehabilitation techniques, or medical concerns.

Popular Online Communities and Support Groups:
- American Stroke Association Support Network

- National Stroke Association Online Support Groups

- Reddit communities such as r/stroke and r/fitness

- Facebook groups focused on stroke recovery, fitness, and wellness

- Health forums and discussion boards on platforms like HealthUnlocked and PatientsLikeMe

By actively engaging in online communities and support groups, individuals undergoing stroke recovery or pursuing fitness goals can find valuable support, information, and encouragement to enhance their journey towards optimal health and well-being.

FURTHER READING AND REFERENCES
Expanding your knowledge and understanding of stroke recovery and fitness can be incredibly beneficial on your journey towards optimal health and well-being. Here are some recommended resources for further reading and references:

1. Books on Stroke Recovery:
   - "Stronger After Stroke: Your Roadmap to Recovery" by Peter G. Levine
   - "My Stroke of Insight: A Brain Scientist's Personal Journey" by Jill Bolte Taylor
   - "The Brain's Way of Healing: Remarkable Discoveries and Recoveries from the Frontiers of Neuroplasticity" by Norman Doidge

2. Academic Journals and Research Articles:
   - Explore peer-reviewed journals such as Stroke, Journal of Stroke and Cerebrovascular Diseases, and Topics in Stroke Rehabilitation for the latest research and advancements in stroke recovery.

- PubMed, Google Scholar, and ResearchGate are valuable resources for accessing scientific articles and research papers related to stroke rehabilitation, exercise physiology, and physical therapy.

3. Websites and Online Portals:
    - American Stroke Association (stroke.org): Provides comprehensive information, resources, and support for stroke survivors, caregivers, and healthcare professionals.
    - National Institute of Neurological Disorders and Stroke (NINDS): Offers information on stroke prevention, treatment, and recovery, along with research updates and educational materials.
    - Mayo Clinic (mayoclinic.org): Features articles, guides, and videos on stroke recovery, rehabilitation exercises, and lifestyle modifications for preventing recurrent strokes.

4. Fitness and Exercise Resources:
    - "ACSM's Guidelines for Exercise Testing and Prescription" by the American College of Sports Medicine: A comprehensive resource for exercise professionals, healthcare providers, and individuals seeking evidence-based guidance on exercise programming.
    - ACE Fitness (acefitness.org): Provides fitness certifications, educational resources, and articles on

exercise physiology, program design, and health coaching.

- IDEA Health & Fitness Association (ideafit.com): Offers continuing education courses, articles, and resources for fitness professionals and enthusiasts.

5. Online Courses and Webinars:
- Coursera (coursera.org) and edX (edx.org): Offer online courses on topics such as stroke rehabilitation, neuroplasticity, exercise science, and physical therapy.
- Webinars hosted by professional organizations, universities, and healthcare institutions provide opportunities to learn from experts and stay updated on the latest research and practices in stroke recovery and fitness.

6. Professional Organizations and Associations:
- American Heart Association (heart.org): Provides resources and educational materials on stroke prevention, treatment, and recovery, along with guidelines for physical activity and exercise.
- National Stroke Association (stroke.org): Offers support groups, educational resources, and advocacy initiatives for stroke survivors, caregivers, and healthcare professionals.

7. Consultation with Healthcare Professionals:
   - Seek guidance and recommendations from healthcare providers, physical therapists, exercise physiologists, and certified fitness professionals for personalized advice and support tailored to your specific needs and goals.

By exploring these additional resources, you can deepen your understanding of stroke recovery, exercise physiology, and wellness practices, empowering yourself to make informed decisions and optimize your health and recovery journey. Remember to critically evaluate information and consult with healthcare professionals for personalized guidance and recommendations.